Elite Personal Training

by Dwayne D. Ivey

Printed in the United States of America

Elite Personal Training

A guide in how to become an elite personal trainer
How to make more than just a living in the fitness industry

by Dwayne D. Ivey

Contents

- Chapter 21-**Men vs. Women in Personal Training** (Who makes a better or more successful trainer?), M*ars &Venus*
- Chapter 22-**Biggest Loser & 24 hour fitness training mentality,** *insanity + danger = motivation*
- Chapter 23-**Firing a client,** *when it's time for the cows to go home*
- Chapter 24-**When a client discontinues training,** (The best protocol to follow with them), *positive separation*
- Chapter 25-**Conclusion,** *you are worthy*

- **Biography**

Acknowledgements

Every project that has merit is never completed by one person alone. I thank my family, colleagues and friends for their suggestions, critiques, editing and support over the course of this effort. In specific, I thank my daughter Camilli for her unbridled patience and love. I also would like to thank, by name, writers Kevin C. Craine (K.C. Craine,) Anthony Bailey and Lupita Villalvazo, medical doctors Riemke Brakema and Yvette LaCoursiere, and longtime friends Bobbi Briseno, Terry LaCoursiere, Miguel Folch contributing photographer, book cover, http://www.miguelfolch.com, info@miguelfolch.com, and Sara Backus, former client (for assistance with some of the copy editing.)

Without the aid of *every* one of these wonderful individuals, this work would not have been completed. To you I bow and say, "Grazie mille!"

Introduction

You want to help people. You have motivation and you are fitness minded. You want to make over $20 per hour and you want to enjoy your work. You may not be sure if you consider personal training to be a profession, but you are willing to try it anyway. Perhaps you are already a personal trainer and you are looking to enhance your skills. These may be some of the thoughts and ideas that have crossed your mind in your pursuit of another career; one that you will use as a stepping stone into another, or maybe you just are looking forward to helping people achieve their fitness goals!

This personal training book will be an insight into the fitness industry and, more specifically, the personal training chaos that you are about to enter into. This guide will be used by both the novice and the fitness directors who manage major national big box fitness clubs.

First, rest assured, personal training *is* a profession. That is, if *you* make it that. Unlike the medical field that has criminal implications if you do not follow the required education curriculum to become a M.D. prior to practicing; personal training requires not much more than you calling yourself a personal trainer and telling people what to do, in essence.

- The field has improved its acceptance as a profession over the last 20 years, but it still has a long way to go. For instance, many local gym managers and owners still hire kids that are right out of high school to be personal trainers. They don't have much more than the Catholic type of send-off before they hit the exercise floor and begin training people and getting straight on the job training (OJT.) If someone gets hurt, "Whoops! Won't do that again." And so it goes.

The American College of Sports Medicine (ACSM) has done the most over the last 20 years to make certifications have standards that are of high professional standard. They are considered to be the Gold Standard of the fitness industry of today. Many professional bodies and certifying agencies watch what the ACSM does to modify their own certification programs and to keep their own standards at a high professional level.

There are over 20 certifications that you can get to be a personal trainer, with most of the certification entities claiming to have national recognition. There are some personal training schools that you can pay to learn at, which are up to six months in duration. You can also find personal training classes at most community colleges that will help you get a nationally recognized certification. Corporate gyms, however, usually require one of between ten to fifteen specific certifications that they recognize nationally and each gym has a different certification acceptance list. There is not much standardization between gyms for what certification is recognized. Gyms do, however, typically have a culture where one certification is recognized above others on the list of national certifications.

There are many items that you need to consider before you jump head first into the pool of chaos known as personal training. This book will serve to both enlighten you and to prepare you for a wonderful career as a professional personal trainer. Pay attention!

For my sons Aaron & Alex and for my daughter Camilli; May you each strive for excellence always.

Also, for every personal trainer and manager; I wish you the utmost success in your business. My goal was to make this an affordable resource for many to enjoy.

Chapter 1

Certifications
Selecting a certification that's right for you

The American College of Sports Medicine (ACSM) is still commonly accepted as the gold standard for certifications in the fitness industry in the United States.

The American Council on Exercise (ACE) process follows closely the recommendations and science found through the ACSM. Personal training manuals and manuals found for the other specializations such as Aerobics Instructor, Clinical Exercise Specialist, and the Advanced Health & Fitness Specialist can be found within most of the national certifications' availability lists.

Teaching aerobics and group classes is a much different focus than one-on-one personal training. In the long run, having one of these alternate and/or advanced certificates will be an advantage for you in your own personal training business.

There are also the following certifications that are widely accepted nationally:

1. American College of Sports Medicine (ACSM)
   http://www.acsm.org/,
2. American Council on Exercise (ACE)
   http://www.acefitness.org/,
3. National Academy of Sports Medicine (NASM)
   http://www.nasm.org/,
4. International Sports Sciences Association (ISSA)
   http://www.issaonline.com/,

5. Aerobics and Fitness Association of America (AFFA)
   http://www.afaa.com/,
6. National Council on Strength and Fitness (NCSF)
   http://www.ncsf.org/ and,
7. American Fitness Professionals and Associates (AFPA)
   http://www.afpafitness.com/

- **Selecting a certification that's right for you**

As you are taking the time to learn about how to become a top trainer and run your own business, you will also need to take the time to research what certification best suits you for your true strengths and passions. Visit each certification and take notes. Write a list of positives and negatives that you see for each. Then, when you are satisfied with the amount of information collected and the certifications that you are comparing, make a decision as to which you like best by closely reviewing your notes.

This is an important part of the process. Do not arbitrarily select a certification because your friend recommended it or because a certain gym requires it for hire. If you are taking your time out to study and pay for the course, take the time now to learn about the subtle, or dramatic, differences between the certifications, their requirements, and their information.

As a part of the selection process, imagine yourself with each certification. Believe it; feel it; then decide if that certification fits you to your core. Does it make you feel good knowing that you have that certification? Or does it make you feel inferior? Does having that certification make you feel like you're missing out on something? For example, if you decide on a certification like ACE, you will find their focus is more aimed at the overall population, not a specific health genre.

NASM, on the other hand, has their focus firmly rooted in training their clients like athletes. If you believe that you want to train a senior like a college athlete, then perhaps NASM will suit your mindset better than that of ACE; which will be more apt to guide you in a more progressive training method for general health. 24 Hour Fitness, the sponsor of the hit show *The Biggest Loser*, in America, for instance, recommends NASM for their trainers. Therefore, their training style correlates close to their personal training certification in the NASM philosophies and methods. For entertainment, *The Biggest Loser* ensures that their trainers treat the participants like athletes, regardless of their age or physical condition.

It's important to feel the emotional passion for your certification because *it will* affect your performance as a personal trainer. If you feel even the slightest bit insecure with your certification or knowledge, you will have difficulty projecting the confidence needed to retain clients or to even obtain them in the first place. Take the time to allow yourself to fully appreciate each certification now, *prior* to investing your precious time and money.

"A teacher affects eternity; he can never tell where his influence stops."

Henry Brooks Adams

Chapter 2

Sales

Personal training is a sales job - techniques that work

Personal training *is* a sales job. I'll say it again; personal training *is* a sales job! You must recognize right at this instant this truth. You will save yourself a lot of heartache over believing that it's not a sales job and believing it is just a job to help people. If you ask any new personal trainer why they became a trainer, you will most likely hear, "I wanted to help people." That is a noble sentiment and a wonderful goal. However, the reality of personal training is that you must be a salesperson and not *just* a do-gooder in order to make a living.

The more people you talk to about personal training, the more you will find out how many people have actually "been" personal trainers. Why aren't they still a trainer? That is the right question to ask. They either got burned out or, like most people, they simply cannot make a living as a personal trainer.

Confidence is a learned leadership behavior. If you do not have confidence, you will not succeed as a top trainer making over $100,000 per year. You might make it as a part-time trainer apart from your "real" career, if that is the case. Confidence is a critical component for the successful personal trainer.

You can begin to build your confidence by simply training as often as you can every day of the week for as long as you can stand it. Being courageous means to stand in the face of your fear and proceed anyway. You must do this regularly in order to train yourself to have confidence. If you find yourself always feeling comfortable in the gym, watch out! Keep putting yourself in situations that make you uncomfortable, in order to grow as a personal trainer. Otherwise, you will be stagnant and soon become trampled over.

Fitness directors and personal training managers want you to succeed. Their bonus depends on it! Their reputation as a club manager does too. These are extremely important ego factors that motivate fitness leaders. For you to be successful as a personal trainer, you will have to initiate and *create* the business. You must be a true pioneer and make something out of nothing. You must interact with the gym members in direct solicitation for their business in order for you to survive! Your paycheck depends on it.

If you simply stand back and think that your education, life experience, athletic or competitive status, or personal training certification are going to get you clients like metal bolts to a magnet, you are wrong and you will sink. Your IQ or education will not earn you clients. They can *help* you get clients and retain those clients; however, you cannot be arrogant and believe they are all you need and that clients should see that. If you do this, you might be successful for a flash in the pan, but you will fizzle out like a Bic lighter.

The best salesman is usually not the one with the most certifications; it's the one that has the most charisma and the most personality. The best salesman is a likable trainer; one that people enjoy being with. Psychology will be discussed in chapter 14.

Furthermore, when making a sale, a seasoned personal trainer knows that their goal is to get the client to ask about purchasing training *before* they have to bring it to the table. This is accomplished by giving a dynamic training session as the *bait* for a client. A personal training session that is both fun and physically taxing for your client, along with informative without being suffocating, is what will elicit the great question, "How much is it to train with you?" When this happens on a regular basis for you as a personal trainer, your client list will be full and both you and your clients will derive great pleasure from the sessions you give.

- The key to obtaining the status of a session selling itself, as a personal trainer, is to fully engross yourself for each minute with your client. Put your blinders on with your client and they will reciprocate by buying sessions from you as long as you're a trainer or until their money runs out, literally.

There are two lists to follow as a new trainer to help get you to the point of "effortless sales." The first list is: **What *to do*** with your client, every session, and the second list is: **What *not* to do** with your client, every session.

What *to do* with your client, every session

- Listen, Be quiet
- Smile
- Ask questions to your client
- Give off an aura of good energy
- Be positive
- Compliment
- Take control
- Be direct
- Be informative
- Give guidance
- Provide the right instruction (visual for visual learners & communicative for audible learners)
- Pay attention to *only* your client
- Keep your hands in front of you, to your sides, or in a place of guidance and support for your client's movement for corrective form placement.

Prior to the session: Do they have any new injuries? Do they have any muscle soreness *today*? How's their energy? When did they eat last? Is there anything that they would really like to work on *today*? Be repetitive. You will keep from injuring your clients if you find out they haven't been eating or sleeping and are sore *prior* to the session. You will also benefit greatly by giving your client what they want, or what they perceive as you paying attention to them, by allowing them to choose an area to focus on during each session. If you never ask them if they would like to really work on something, they will think that you are not listening to their needs. Ultimately, you will lose that client.

During the session: What exercises did they do between days with you? Did they follow your advice? Did they skip a workout? Why? Ask how their companion or spouse is doing. Ask how their family is doing. When you accompany a good workout with empathetic and caring questions & communication, your client will leave not only feeling great physically, but also feeling mental relief and stress reduction too.

What *not* to do with your client, every session

- Talk incessantly
- Talk about yourself
- Talk about your problems
- Give too much information about your personal life
- During weight movement, do not talk about anything *except* the work involved or tips (weight movement is the critical stage of the workout. If you are slack and injury occurs, you will be negligent in your duty and you will be held liable, regardless of the insurance that you or the gym carries)
- Lean on machines (NEVER do this!)
- Communicate with other employees, trainers, or members (no casual conversation!)

- Do not lead your client like a horse (walk beside them like a person, not in front of them)

The *walk-away* technique

There is a widely known phenomenon in the personal training world. It is known as the *walk-away* technique.

Consider this, have you ever walked into a car dealership? What was your feeling like? Did you feel like a rabbit about to be pounced on by a pack of coyote? Or, did you feel like carnage on the road about to be scavenged by birds of prey? If so, you're not alone.

When people *feel* like they are being *sold* something, they turn "off." You lose even the potential for a sale. The moment disappears suddenly, just like a cloud in the sky might. It is your duty as an expert personal trainer to put exercise members at ease and be welcoming and inviting; not threatening or pushy.

Most seasoned exercise veterans can spot a trainer on the prowl like a boxer can see an opening for a punch in a boxing match. These self-proclaimed fitness know-it-alls will chat it up with you and snub you after wasting loads of your time. And, you may not even realize that you are wasting your time, you might think you are getting on their good side to maybe one day be able to solicit a sale from them!

For seasoned exercisers, and for new members alike, you may need to execute the *walk-away* technique.

This technique is a specific, and brief, free service that you give to the member. It's usually unsolicited and can be given in just a few seconds time. You give a great service to your members and you save yourself a ton of potentially wasted time with someone who wants to do just that with you; waste your time, or gain information that should be paid for.

How to execute the *walk-away* technique

- An example:

  You are an expert at picking out bad form on exercise equipment. You observe a member doing something bad and potentially dangerous. You walk up to the member (*after* they have completed the set, NEVER during weight movement!)

  You introduce yourself (they probably don't know you) and you ask them if you could give them a free tip. They say, "yes." You then give a succinct definition of the exercise that they are doing and what muscles are involved by saying, "I'm sure you already know this but…" This gives you the momentary credibility that you need to give your advice (they will most likely already know what muscles they are working, not always, but typically.)

  You then describe to them good form for the exercise they are doing, or you demonstrate it briefly. This should all be done within the amount of time they are resting between sets, not as an over explanation that interrupts their workout. You then ask them to perform the next set with their newly learned tip in place. After a few reps, you say, "Great! Looks good, keep up the good work!", and you simply *walk-away*. It's that easy. That member, and every member eavesdropping, will appreciate your service and this type of technique will yield future training sessions sold that seem to come "out of the blue." Many times, training sessions will be bought by an *observer*, not just the member you gave the service to!

The Body Fat Table

Some of the greatest tools available for a pioneering personal trainer inside of a big box gym are simply tables & chairs. Confidence will only be gained with direct and regular interaction with the gym members. Instead of waiting for your gym manager to send you clients or to hover over you while you attempt to cold sell the members by direct sales on the gym floor, known as "prospecting," a proven approachable sales method is The Body Fat Table.

If you regularly set up a table and two chairs in a conspicuous place in the walkway or near the water fountains in your gym, you will sell personal training packages and/or nutritionals to members that you initiate conversation with or to members that initiate the conversation with you! For new trainers especially, this can help bolster self-confidence and assist in finding the weaknesses in your knowledge base and it will improve your ability to answer fitness questions from inquiring gym members. Instead of pacing the gym floor looking like a lion scouting his next zebra fill, you will not be as intimidating as you stand, and not sit, near your table and chairs with your Omron body fat electronic impedance device. On your table you should also include copies of free health tips that you put together or that you copied from your certifications' newsletters, etc. If you have funding, or use your own money, you can get a few helium balloons from the local party store for a few dollars which will help draw attention to your table.

Members will ask you a multitude of questions and even the gym rats will stop and strike up conversation to test your knowledge and to "show off" how much they know, many times quoting articles from Muscle & Fitness and similar publications.
This table is a proving ground for you to build your confidence, make sales, and learn the areas of your expertise that need additional focus. Because of the proven sales success of this method, while I was a personal training manager, this table was a daily requirement that my staff were required to man during morning and afternoon peak and non-peak hours. Even at 2 p.m. in the afternoon on any given Tuesday, a $1000 + personal training package would be regularly sold by my staff,

or by me, while there appeared to be no potential sale in sight. The table works, use it.

Demeanor is crucial while at this table. This is not a time for you to talk to the membership representatives about your weekend. This is not the time to sit down, kick your heels back, and look like you're about to fall asleep. Be attentive. Smile. Simply, freely and lightly ask each member that walks by your table if they would like a "free" body fat test. You will hear some pretty interesting answers, but many will stop.

Once you have taken the sixty seconds to input the member's information into the electronic impedance device, and they are gripping it awaiting their results, this is a magical time in space that you have to ask the member about their last training experience or to offer a complimentary session with you. Of course, ideally, you will sit down with this member and give them a brief nutrition consultation or analyze their current workout regime with them. With practice, you will go from asking the member if they want a free body fat test to swiping their credit card for a personal training package purchase within ten to thirty minutes of your time. If you sell even just one package per week for your hour of time every other day, your client list will be bulging quickly. And, whenever you need more clients, don't forget about The Body Fat Table! It will surprise you.

The Front Desk

This is a direct personal training sales approach that a lot of gyms that have motivated fitness managers put into practice. Depending on your gym, you will have a variety of ways for a member to "check-in" for their daily workout. Typically, you will see on the computer screen, on the employee side of the counter, the member's account information, including their name.

A lot of managers push their new trainers to the front desk to give them exposure and to solicit clients directly. The front desk is a tricky entity. Most members entering the gym are customarily in a hurry or they are just not interested in striking up a friendly conversation as they just enter the gym. I wouldn't suggest you attempt to hard sell any member from the front desk as they are entering the facility. Instead, be a warm, smiling welcome for them to see, and mention to them that you are available for any exercise or nutrition questions that they have or may think of during their work out. The idea is to make contact in a friendly manner, do not be aggressive or intimidating by looking like you are desperate for a sale. Be sincere and genuine. I understand why managers send new employees to the front desk, but usually they are left there to fend for themselves with little or no guidance from the manager in what to do or in how to act. It can be very awkward to a new trainer in a way that they begin to dread arriving to the gym because all their manager is going to do is send them to the front desk.

The front desk is a great place for exposure and for digging for rapport with members but focus your attention on members that need assistance or that are leaving the facility. Members that are leaving the gym are typically feeling better than they arrived due to their physiological response to whatever activity they did inside the gym. The barriers that were initially in place with the member upon their entry have dissipated like a late morning fog and you now have a door to knock on instead of a steel wall keeping you out.

The front desk is also a way of waving the flag, so to speak. Identifying the presence of the personal training staff and having them available is important. Having a personal trainer at the front desk is always helpful for members in need. And, many times, the personal trainer that is at the front desk that walks away with a member in need, will ultimately be savvy enough to next be sitting in an office setting up a personal training appointment that is complimentary or he will be giving away some other type of advice. Either way, this is a service that will also yield sales. The key is to not be pushy yet you must also have the ulterior motive of setting up a free personal training session at least. This goes back to the basic sales principle, if you do not ask for a sale you will not get it. You must have the intention of setting up an appointment, but you can't badger them into it. There's a fine line that you will be able to navigate the more that you put yourself out there and the more confidence that you gain from this type of exposure.

The front desk is just one more of the sales efforts that a personal trainer can take advantage of, but you must be alert and not lazy. Otherwise, your efforts will be fruitless.

"Real integrity is doing the right thing, knowing that nobody's going to know whether you did it or not."

Oprah Winfrey

Chapter 3

Money/Income
How you can make over 100k

How much money can you expect to make as a personal trainer? Do you think $15 per hour is amazing? Can you make $50 or more per hour? Do you believe that you can make over $100,000 gross in a year for your work as a personal trainer?

If you focus your efforts, you certainly can make over $100,000 per year in income. That is the good news. On the other hand, if you are timid and you are not fully engrossed in the fitness world, you can easily make less than the poverty level in income as a personal trainer. There is a clear line of distinction between successful professional personal trainers, and personal trainers who will not make it. This distinction has already been mentioned: confidence.

In the beginning, you will probably work for a gym. That is how most celebrity trainers begin; in the school of hard-knocks one-on-one in front of new exercise members in a gym atmosphere. Your salary will most likely be the minimum wage plus any sessions that you service for an additional $7-15 per hour.

As you gain experience, and as you fulfill that particular gym's requirements to advance, you will typically earn more in pay. Ultimately, you can be working full time 30-50 hours per week as a trainer with 20 plus clients. You can make up to $45 per hour for training sessions serviced in corporate gyms as a professional personal trainer. As a trainer that owns his own business, you can realistically make up to $80 per hour, gross. If you include special services, in addition to your training, such as professional training PNF or AIS, or massage therapy, then you can realistically make an income of up to $150 per hour. When it comes to fitness, people will invest their money to feel better, get better looks, or to try to extend their life.

The greatest fear new personal trainers have is approaching an individual and asking for their money. In sales it's called, "Asking for the sale." It's simple; if you do not ask for their money, you cannot get it.

Many trainers will choke up in fear and become paralyzed and panic at the moment of sale. They will lose the sale at the very moment they could have made it had they approached that moment with confidence and excitement. This is why good sales managers will have new personal trainers shadow them (the act of watching sales occur with the sales manager making the sale) or they will make the new employee shadow an experienced trainer during the first few days to first few weeks of their employment *prior* to allowing them to attempt their first sale. If the gym is desperate for income, or the management philosophy is, "We give them baptism by fire" then you may be out on the floor by yourself your first day without guidance. That happened to me, it can happen to you. (Ultimately, I became a personal training manager and then owned my own studio that grossed over 100k annually.)

The gym will terminate your employment if after your "probationary period" you do not keep clients or if you do not make sales. The gym cannot simply afford to pay you if you're not producing. Their existence depends on sales. It begins with membership sales which is a corporate gym's main source of revenue. Then the gym depends on the income from personal training and the retail department. Personal training revenue is the single source of "free" and real revenue in a gym. The entire revenue gained by the personal training department will pay executive bonuses and manager bonuses after expenses, in most settings. Therefore, if you are not producing, you can bet you will not work there for more than a few months.

Trainers that *do not do* sales, and expect to make an income anyhow, will not survive as a personal trainer for more than six months. So if you are seeking a career change and you are currently making a great salary, do not abandon your job to become a personal trainer exclusively, until after you get your feet wet and train part time to see how you really like the experience and the job. In personal training it is easy to fantasize that the job is easy with good hours and great pay, but the reality is not that way at all in the beginning.

Once you gain experience through hundreds of appointments and thousands of successful training hours, you will begin to enjoy the benefit of being a professional personal trainer. The fantasy, then, is not completely unrealistic; it *is* possible.

"If money is your hope for independence you will never have it. The only real security that a man will have in this world is a reserve of knowledge, experience, and ability."

Henry Ford

Chapter 4

Corporate gyms
Working for the big boys

Entering into the corporate gym industry can be both a daunting task and exciting. You must realize that you will have to be persistent as a personal trainer, especially in the beginning.

At the very beginning, you will be placed under the microscope by the managers and other employees. If any of the managers do not like you, you will not get hired-it's that easy. Your certifications *do* give you a certain amount of credibility as to your interest in being a trainer, however. It doesn't mean you *have to* begin a personal training job with a certification though. Most intelligent gym managers will occasionally deviate from their policies and guidelines of hiring *only* certified trainers.

If you do not have a certification, it is much easier for a gym manager to tell you to come back when you have one, rather than telling you they are not interested in hiring you. If you then later go back with the certification in hand, they can just say they are not hiring; rather than tell you that they don't want you on their team. There are fears of lawsuits and of hurting your feelings, even from the best managers. If you encounter this type of situation, it's best and easiest to make a mental note to not apply at that gym again until new management has taken over-which *will* occur at some time in the future, this you can take to the bank. Management at gyms has a pretty high turn-over rate. Either the manager will get promoted, moved, or they simply will take a position with a different company. Every individual gym, even gyms of the same corporation, will have a different management style within its doors. While they may share a common district or regional manager, a particular gym's energy will flow directly from that gym's general manager and personal training or sales manager.

The hierarchy of a corporate gym will typically be something like this:

- President/CEO
- Senior Vice-President
- Vice President(s)
- Regional Manager(s)
- District Manager(s)
- General Manager(s)
- Sales Manager(s), Fitness Director(s) (personal training managers)
- Personal Trainer, Aerobics Instructor, Pilates Instructor, Yoga Instructor, Cycling Instructor
- Cleaning staff, equipment maintenance, kids' club employees

A corporation will have an agenda for their personal training manager and team. You can expect to undergo some "in-house" training as an attempt to direct your training philosophy and methods. In most cases, you will need to follow their approach, regardless of your certification, in order to remain employed by them. This is not the case if you are an independent contractor where most state laws dictate specifically that a business owner cannot direct the *way* you train or tell you what methods to use. Every gym operates in its own manner and it will be up to you to figure out if their philosophies, or the contract, are ones that you will be in agreement with. Do not alter your core training philosophies or beliefs for another. You will be a much happier and successful trainer if you find the gym that will be the best *fit* for you.

At some gyms you will find that you may not agree with certain elements of their philosophy. If this happens don't fret. Every gym will have something that may not appeal to you. You may just have to accept it. For example, many gyms *require* you to sell nutrition supplements. In addition to your quota as a personal trainer (yes, you *will* have a quota to fulfill!), you will also have a quota to sell a certain amount of supplements per month. While you will receive a hefty commission for doing so, perhaps selling supplements is not a part of your belief system. These are also elements of consideration.

Professional trainers usually get their start in a big box gym like 24 Hour Fitness, Bally Total Fitness, LA Fitness, or the like. After working for several years, trainers begin to realize that they are paying a hefty fee to these gyms for the benefit of using their equipment and space. Some of these trainers become managers and are happy with that status. The other intelligent trainers, now with experience and a full client list, will evaluate how much money they are "giving" back to the gym from their paychecks for these elements. Then, they will either decide to settle and remain indefinitely with the corporation, or they will leave and begin their own private personal training studio. They will realize that they can make more money and not have to deal with the corporate mandates and procedures-they can train *their* way and officially be their own boss.

Most corporations make you sign an agreement saying that you won't leave and take your clients with them. In spite of this, this is how most personal training studios begin-with the professional trainer leaving the corporate world to begin their own business and by taking the clients they obtained with them while at that corporation.

The trainer's clients will simply follow their trainers anywhere, and probably pay less at the new studio while their trainer makes more per hour for the same service. This is a regular occurrence and one that drives district managers crazy because it directly affects their income when a professional successful trainer not only leaves their gym, but also takes that income away with them. Sure the corporations could go to court and win the case against these trainers most of the time, but the reality is that it would tie up too much money in revenue to pursue each trainer that did this. Ultimately, they save money by not taking these trainers to court; but instead by just deciding to cut their losses and work with the business that they have left.

In the end, corporations are a great starting point for you, the new personal trainer. The guidance and experience that you will receive as a personal trainer in a big box gym will give you the backbone, confidence, and training that you will need to be a successful professional trainer.

You will get the added benefit of working with difficult managers, employees, and clients alike. This will give you resiliency or it will knock you out of the industry. Either way, you win.

Aside from having the immediate benefit of potential clients available to you in a large gym; a desirable element of working for a corporation are the potential medical & dental benefits that can be derived by working for them. You also don't have to think about taking care of taxes in any other way than any other employee would have to. When you work for yourself, you have to pay additional taxes.

"To survive, men and business and corporations must serve."

John H. Patterson

Chapter 5

Local gyms
The good and the bad

In your city you will have four basic types of personal training opportunities, as a trainer:

1) Big box gym,
2) Local gym,
3) In-home training, and
4) Your own training studio.

There *are* additional positions, obviously, such as working with: universities, Pro sports teams, and medical doctors. These jobs usually come after a great deal of experience and after finding your niche, however, and not as a brand new personal trainer.

Local gyms operate a whole lot differently than the big boys do. The first difference can be seen in the gym itself. The gym is typically owned and operated by a local businessman. These gyms tend to tailor their activities and staff depending on the desire of the community, not in a manner that is dictated from someone sitting in an office in Los Angeles or New York. Their methods can result in the gym taking on an atmosphere of muscle heads or sweaty gym rats; or one of a friendly neighborhood gym, depending on the owner's personal vision for that gym. Many times these gyms will not be able to afford a general manager or a fitness director's usual salary, so they will settle for less experienced individuals to keep their overhead down and their profits up. This does not help benefit you as a trainer looking to get quality experience.

If the manager was hired because he was a friend of the owner, or because they are what the owner could afford; beware. You may be excited that they are going to employ you initially, but in the long run you will lose out on the seniority benefits and quality sales instruction that you could have potentially received from a bigger establishment.

You can identify these types of gyms easily by their hiring practice. Many times you will find that they do not require you to have a national personal training certification at all. Instead, they will *train* you their way and give you their "certification" and bless you as a certified personal trainer; which is deceptive practice and not good for the fitness industry as a whole.

Then, when you leave that gym to work for another, their certification will do you as much good as knowing *that* gym's motto-it will be useless and you will most likely have learned a lot of bad training habits that will inhibit your progress toward being a professional and successful personal trainer.

If you live in a small city, it might be impossible for you to avoid working for a gym like this. In that case, you will need to enhance yourself in sales and in your personal training abilities. You can do this by obtaining advanced certifications such as the Clinical Exercise Specialist certification. You can also seek better sales approaches and methods either by attending your local community college and university, or by taking online courses to develop your skills.

Take caution with the benefits available from a local gym too. Typically they are less apt to offer medical and dental benefits, not to mention 401K or a similar type of retirement plan.

"The resistance that you fight physically in the gym and the resistance that you fight in life can only build a strong character."

Arnold Schwarzenegger

Chapter 6

Private studios

Freedom with a catch: overhead

Professional trainers that remain dependent on their clients' income to survive tend to be intelligent individuals. If you become successful as a trainer, you will contemplate your own exodus from the corporate atmosphere at some point during your career.

For many, having a private personal training studio is the epitome of success in personal training; owning your own business. For some, it's not even a consideration as they have settled and are comfortable working for someone.

If you choose to venture away from the comforts of the corporate world and begin your own studio, you will need a regular clientele to maintain your overhead and keep you fed. If you are like most of the trainers and you bring the bulk of your clients with you from the big box gym, then this element will not be an issue for you; your income source is already flowing and you just have to sustain it.

On the other hand, if you are a new trainer and you have the capital or financial backing to begin a start-up personal training studio of your own, you will have to take on the incredible task of obtaining a client base by marketing and solicitation, in addition to maintaining the responsibilities of owning a studio. These responsibilities include: the lease, electric, insurance, water, and the other building expenses that come with ownership or as stipulated in a lease agreement.

If you are planning on opening up your own personal training studio, you will be looking out for your best interests if you gain necessary personal training experience and skills by working for someone first. In this way you can also cater to your clients in a way you otherwise would not be able to relate. You will get the benefit of being able to have a contrast between the big box gym's philosophies and management, and that of your own private studio.

Creating a business plan for your personal training studio is a logical first step *prior* to fully committing to the idea and allocating all of your resources and time. The mere act of becoming aware of all of the facts about owning a business in your state might be enough to dissuade you from beginning a process that you otherwise may not be prepared for. Awareness, too, can act as a catalyst to propel you into ownership of your own private studio quicker than you had anticipated.

After expenses, a professional personal trainer that owns a studio can expect a net profit of at least $30,000 per year after overhead and taxes with the right preparation. This is with the expectation of working at least part time hours of 25-30 hours per week. If you thrive off of working long hours constantly throughout the day (many trainers do) you can almost double your net expectation.

Hiring employees at your personal training studio is yet another option. If you own a facility, it might behoove you to employ at least one other trainer to share the space with you. You create the contract (independent contractor) agreement with the trainer and, in exchange for their work; you receive either rent or a percentage of their sales while training at your studio. For those with great facilitation and management abilities, this may be a very lucrative route to pursue. Each state has different requirements from business owners that hire independent contractors. Be sure to consult your local laws to ensure compliance or you may be paying fines for violating them, or worse-you could be sued.

"Dealing with people is probably the biggest problem you face, especially if you are in business. Yes, and that is also true if you are a housewife, architect or engineer."

Dale Carnegie

Chapter 7

In-home training
The traveling salesman

During the interview process with a gym, there is always the point where you are talking directly with the hiring official. It is during this interview that you must give full disclosure and let them know that you *also* do in-home training *and* that you have clients. If you do not do this, you may be setting yourself up for a conflict of interest if you later decide to do in-home training as the company will consider your training a conflict of interest to your employment and they may terminate you. If you go into the employment with their knowledge of your outside activity, you will not encounter this issue as they will have given their "ok" for this activity *in spite* of their employment of you.

After gaining experience in gyms, you can elect to do *only* in-home training as this limits your overhead expenditures and allows you great liberty to travel and be "outside" throughout the week as you drive from one client's home to another. You can have a full array of equipment that you keep in your "mobile gym" or in your vehicle to accommodate situations when your clients do not have enough equipment or if they do not have a home gym available.

There are a few personal trainers that do begin by simply training friends and later become in-home trainers right off, rather than working for a gym. This is not the norm, but it could be what suits you.

Referrals, regardless of how you start or where you end up in the personal training business, are one of the most important sources of your business that you will ever have. Your current clients will refer others to you if they like you and if your services provide results.

Referrals will get you to the point of having a waiting list a lot faster than advertising and marketing will. You can attempt to begin your career by starting with in-home training; however, you are losing out on a lot of incredible gym training experience and enhancement if you do.

"It's just such a freeing thing to set these great challenges for yourself, to travel, to learn more about the world, to just go out there and get crazy and get free and get strong."

Angelina Jolie

Chapter 8

Niches
You must have one to be successful

After several months or several years of servicing personal training appointments and sessions, you will find yourself gravitating toward a specific group of individuals more than others, if you don't already.

This is an important element for you as a trainer known as a niche. This specificity of training will be what separates you and your unique abilities in the realm of personal training. This specificity of training will be what gets you to have a waiting list and it will draw you referrals from other health professionals and your co-workers. For example, if you are the best at what you do with seniors in your area, who do you think your co-worker will refer to when they realize that they are in over their head? When a medical doctor needs a specialist for his patient, who do you think he will feel confident in giving a recommendation to?

Professionals appreciate other professionals having a passion, and they appreciate the extra skills and knowledge they have in specific areas of health. There are countless specialties available in fitness when considering personal training. Personal training is much more than simply training the obese or fat people, to lose weight. Personal training involves working with athletes, pregnancy (pre/post,) seniors, children, cancer patients, heart patients, spinal injury clients, stroke patients, and with clients with knee and/or other joint injuries or limitations. Each specialty requires additional knowledge, skills, and abilities in order for you to safely and effectively work with these clients.

When you narrow down your scope to working mostly, *or only*, with a certain group, you begin to separate yourself from the common trainer and you begin to become accepted as a specialist with a certain group. Over a period of time, of months or years, you develop accepted expert status with that niche group of individuals.

Becoming a specialist is much like planting a fruit tree. You first begin with a seedling, then over a period of time, the leaves begin to develop and eventually you have your fruit that is ripe and ready for picking. This is the point of having obtained as much business as you *want* to handle, and perhaps of having that much desired waiting and referral list.

When becoming a personal trainer, you want to begin to think about what groups of people you are both most passionate about working with and that you are most successful working with.

You may begin your career believing that you want to work with completely healthy adults and athletes and after a few years you may discover that your client list is full of senior citizens and cancer patients.

You must be both open to the idea that your specific niche is potentially different than what you think it is going to be and you must be willing to modify your paradigm as the work presents itself. Otherwise you may miss the boat and be left wondering why you struggle to keep a client roster or why renewing training with clients is arduous when it's time.

"I've had to work very hard, and I don't really have a category or fit into any niche, so each time I come out with a new record, it's like, I'm a new guy."

Lenny Kravitz

Chapter 9

Retirement
Planning and resources

Retirement is all about planning. It's not about being in a certain job or career. How many times have you heard the story about so and so dying and leaving millions to such and such charity? This is always echoed by the media spouting something like, "How can this be? He was a train conductor!", or, "She may have lived frugally as a waitress, but she gave millions!"

As a professional personal trainer, you have the opportunity to sock away a fortune, too. You don't have to be a Registered Nurse (RN) or work for the city, state or federal government to "get the benefits." The fact of the matter is that you have to take time out to research what retirement option you choose to plan for. If you do not plan for retirement, you will not have a retirement plan-it's that easy.

The difference between a hospital, the government, or a big company and you is that they do the thinking for you. They tell you what their retirement plan is and you either agree with it and you contribute more into it than what they do, or you don't. It is a complete misconception that you must work for a particular company in order to get a good retirement. The fact is that you must take time out and learn about this on your own, which you should do anyway regardless of whether you work for yourself or for someone.

The United States Government has had a worthwhile program in place for a few years now, though it has gone seemingly unnoticed by most people. It is highly misunderstood, as well.

- Evaluate the U.S. Department of the Treasury's *Health Savings Accounts (HSA's)* for yourself. There are a multitude of benefits from this plan. Their mission statement reads, "Health Savings Accounts (HSAs) were created by the Medicare bill signed by President Bush on December 8, 2003 and are designed to help individuals save for future qualified medical and retiree health expenses on a tax-free basis." Tax free! Now *that* is what I'm talking about! You can gain easy access to this information online at: http://www.ustreas.gov/offices/public-affairs/hsa/.

The fact of the matter is that you are in control of your retirement, regardless of what your status is in life. You must save and invest wisely. You must live below your means. There are financial gurus and books available at your local bookstore to educate you on how to plan for your retirement. Don't be lazy, go buy these resources and become educated. Then, take the time and exert the effort to implement these practices into your life along with your newfound career as a professional exercise expert. Otherwise, you will find yourself wanting to change careers after ten or fifteen years for something you perceive as "more secure," like a career of a RN or government employee.

If you are not lazy, you will have a great retirement following your tenure as a career exercise professional. If you allow the world to dictate your retirement, the opposite will be your lot.

"Choose a work that you love and you won't have to work another day."

Confucius

Chapter 10

Benefits
They're just misunderstood

Like retirement, benefits are often misunderstood. Just because your employer may now *provide* you with a great health plan, does not mean that is the best thing for you.

What do you think all of the small business owners in the United States do for health care? Do you think they pay the high premiums for insurance costs for plans like Blue Cross/Blue Shield or any of the multitudes of other carriers available? Sometimes, yes they do. Other times, they do not. Instead, the others pay out of pocket as the need arises.

I am certainly not advocating that you go without health insurance, but what I am advocating is that you become knowledgeable in what your *real* options are. For example, did you know that hospitals and doctors give *different* rates for people that pay out of pocket on their own, versus what their rates are for insurance companies? It stands to reason why insurance is so expensive-when insurance pays, they *really* pay! Ultimately, it is we, the consumer, which pays by both the insurance companies' gouging and the abuse by hospitals and industries everywhere that overcharge insurance companies for service and/or product.

Take a look at your hospital bill the next time you go. Does an 80mg aspirin really cost over four dollars for one? If you pay out of pocket for your emergency and regular annual physical checkups, many times you will save money over the long haul, compared to throwing your money at an insurance company every month for the "just in case" factor. This also relates to the HSA's mentioned in the retirement chapter. The money you put into a HSA is yours, not an insurance executive's. Take the time to do your research for what your real costs are, or what they could be for you and your family's needs. Then, make a decision that is custom made for you and your family. People generally don't want to think about the specifics and the details involved with selecting a route for health care or other benefits. You will find, though, that if you do this, you will not only be informed, you will also gain confidence with the knowledge obtained.

"Opportunity can benefit no man who has not fitted himself to seize it and use it. Opportunity woos the worthy, shuns the unworthy. Prepare yourself to grasp opportunity, and opportunity is likely to come your way. It is not so fickle, capricious and unreasoning as some complain."

B. C. Forbes

Chapter 11

Health care team, what it is
The best health care in town

A health care team is what you can be a part of. It's about having the best system in place for you and for your family. You will be on the service side as a professional personal trainer. You will provide a key role in the lives of every one of your clients. It is imperative that you come to terms with what your role is as the exercise expert, and how you can best serve your client. It is your responsibility to do this, and your clients will appreciate you all the more for it. Do not be passive, you are the exercise expert!

A health care team can be all or a selection of some of the following:

- Family Practitioner (M.D.)
- Osteopathic Physician (D.O.)
- Registered Nurse (R.N.)
- Pediatrician (M.D.)
- Chiropractor (D.C.)
- Surgeon (M.D.)
- Naturopathic Doctor (N.D.)
- Registered Dietitian (R.D.)
- Physical Therapist (P.T.)
- Exercise Physiologist
- Clinical Exercise Specialist
- Health & Fitness Specialist
- Certified Personal Trainer
- Acupuncturist (L Ac.)
- Certified/Licensed Massage Therapist

Your national personal trainer certification likely covers the importance of communication with your client's doctor, to a fault. In the real world in any gym, you will not have any contact with your client's doctor *unless* you force the issue. The fact is that *if you must* have an exercise clearance from a potential client, you will not sell the personal training package that day without one. Therefore, you will not be servicing that client and you will not get paid.

Most often, you will get a statement from your client to the effect of, "I'm fine, and my doctor says I'm fine." You will then proceed to train this individual. You will even get this statement from clients that *are* doctors! National certification bodies are strict on their policies, and to your adherence to those policies, for you to remain certified by them (for liability reasons.) The truth is, though, that you *will not* ordinarily complete the Physical Activities Readiness Questionnaire (PARQ) that they are adamant that you must do *every time* you give an exercise consultation. You really should fill one out for your own protection, however.

Since every person is unique and with issues related specifically to them, it stands to reason that every health care team, or circle of care, will be different depending on the client.

For example, you may have one client that the circle of care will begin with their family practitioner. They may be seeing a registered dietitian as recommended by their doctor. They may also be seen by the doctor's registered nurse and by a physical therapist. Perhaps the doctor is now recommending an exercise regimen for her patient, your client. You are then added to the circle of care.

In this example the circle of care, the health care team, for this client is: M.D., R.D., R.N., P.T., and certified personal trainer.

- Note: P.T. is reserved legally for only physical therapists, not for personal trainers.

As the exercise expert, it will be up to you to coordinate communication between each of your client's team members. Ideally this communication path would be facilitated by your client's family practitioner (M.D.), however, since most doctors are strapped for time, this will not be the case.

In order to facilitate this communication, you may need to spend a considerable amount of time getting to know these specific individuals, which may prove to be a difficult, if not impossible, task. Your national certification will give you protocol for obtaining necessary information from your client's doctor, including forms that can be signed by their doctor identifying their exercise clearance. Due to privacy laws, it is imperative that you follow legal channels for obtaining information and by first getting permission from your client.

The circle of care is an ideal situation for any individual, you included, for optimum health care & maintenance.

- Imagine: Your doctor, nurse, dietitian, physical therapist, *and* your personal trainer all on-board together for *your* benefit! They communicate openly about how they have worked to improve your health and they share ideas and voice concerns with each other. Ultimately, each professional will take notes and take into consideration different facets of each of the expert's observations and experiences with you. Your health care team gives each other recommendations based on their skills and you end up with a completely customized health care approach for the most important person in your life; you!

Does that extent of care sound like fantasy to you? If so, it shouldn't. I was a participant, for example, in a concierge health care environment where this scenario played out for me for nearly two years with my clients, until I left.

In a typical gym setting, you may not need to go to this extent of service with your clients, but there are times when you should. You will have to gain hands-on experience to be able to detect when it is critical that you do this for your client. You can get by for an entire career and not ever give this type of service to a client. If you care about the status of the fitness industry, and if you care about giving the best service possible as an exercise professional, don't you think that it is important that you aim for this type of advanced service? You owe it to your clients to give them the best service you can. They are, after all, paying $60-$90 on average for every session with you! What kind of service would you expect if you paid someone that much money for one hour of time? Take the time to get to know your clients, and their health care team. Be a part of the team, not just an outside observer!

"The physician should look upon the patient as a besieged city and try to rescue him with every means that art and science place at his command."

Alexander of Tralles

Chapter 12

Quotas
The ugly truth

There are two types of trainers: Those that don't mind quotas, and those that despise quotas.

Successful trainers are those that don't mind having a specific dollar amount of sales to make each month as their quota.

New and/or unconfident trainers are the trainers that are afraid of quotas.

As mentioned in the Sales chapter, you are a salesman as a personal trainer. Every gym that will hire you expects that you perform sales.

If you are not a fan of selling, don't fret. You can focus your energy into giving great quality service and your training can sell itself. Many times, too, your sales manager or fitness director will be willing to *close* the sale for you, provided that you give great service. With time, you will find that you will become comfortable with the sales aspect of personal training and quotas won't even make you blink.

You will be required, at minimum, to sell personal training sessions and packages. You may be required to fulfill a supplement sales quota along with perhaps a membership sign-up quota or even miscellaneous quotas that pop up from time to time from corporate headquarters.

"In this business, by the time you realize you're in trouble, it's too late to save yourself. Unless you're running scared all the time, you're gone."

Bill Gates

Chapter 13

Supplements
It's about profit

Many personal trainers do not like being forced to sell nutritional supplements or other items-they just want to train! Be prepared, if you go to work for a big box gym, to sell *more* than just personal training. You will be expected to be on-board with *their* program and philosophy, or they will not hire you.

Gyms make their money in several different ways. As previously mentioned, selling supplements, in addition to personal training, is big business and they earn a lot of profit by enforcing quotas on supplements. The supplement industry is a billion dollar a year business and you may find yourself being a part of it. Typically, you will earn a nice bonus on your checks for selling supplements in a gym. You will have to learn about the specifics in the gym that you are applying for to see what their requirements are and what their commissions are for selling supplements.

You should also take into consideration what your national certification's policies are with regards to supplements. Most will not advocate the use of any supplement. Most will not allow you to make recommendations of supplements to your clients without breaking their policies and in effect excluding you from their liability protection. Be aware of, and sensitive to, what the rules are for your certification and compare those to what the gym is requiring you to do.

Often, you will be the one left hanging out to dry if something happens to your client. The gym will still be in the lawsuit, but *you* were the one making the recommendation and against your certification's policies, so where is your protection? It's in your judgment and use of common sense. I understand the need to work and gyms have a tendency to put you in between a rock and a hard place with specific regards to enforcing quotas on supplement sales. Be aware, and make decisions that will protect you, not leave you standing alone.

"For every minute you are angry you lose sixty seconds of happiness."

Ralph Waldo Emerson

Chapter 14

Psychology
Your real job

Psychology is arguably the most important factor involved in being a personal trainer. While you are most likely not a licensed doctor or therapist, most of your interaction with your clients will have elements that a keen professional trainer will be able to recognize. These elements are mostly emotional in nature. They include a person's: confidence, self-worth, self-esteem, body image, family issues, marital problems, job challenges, and other sensitive psychological factors.

Though every professional personal trainer will have the skills to communicate with their clients and their issues, most of the national personal trainer certifications do little more than touch on the topic. They do not expand on psychology and they fail to prepare you for such crucial and intimate encounters. I implore you to seek out community college and/or university classes that are specifically geared to human psychology. You may not want to be a therapist, doctor, or shrink, but the fact is that as a personal trainer you will spend many quality hours with your client. Often, you will find that your client spends more time with you than their spouses or companions.

You, their personal trainer, are in a sensitive and unbiased position and therefore you become a safe sounding board and sponge. Since your sessions are private and personal, your client begins to trust you and they often begin to depend on you for emotional support too. For these reasons it is important for you to set boundaries when it comes to professionalism and interaction. You can be a safe and unbiased resource for them to feel comfortable around but be careful. You are not a licensed therapist and you should not be making recommendations, and you should especially not be giving prescriptions or you can be held legally liable and accountable for your actions. If you have a basic understanding of psychology through some of the courses recommended above, you will be better prepared to handle situations that will arise and you will readily identify when you should make a professional recommendation to a psychologist or other health care team member. If you are ignorant, you are doing a disservice to your client and setting yourself up for potentially life changing events.

Do yourself a favor and do not play psychologist. Be your client's personal trainer, their professional resource for physical activity and nutrition guidance. As a professional and knowledgeable personal trainer, you will acknowledge the need for outside mental help and you, having gained your client's trust, are in a wonderful position to make recommendations for seeing a therapist or counselor. You may make a few mistakes in the beginning, but with practice you will be tactful and respectful and make professional recommendations without insulting your client.

- Remember: Your client spends hours upon hours with you week after week. You are a leader in their world. What you have to say has an impact in their lives. Be courteous and empathetic, but do not overstep your bounds or scope of duty as a personal trainer. You owe it to your client, and yourself, to make the professional recommendations as you see fit. Once you make a recommendation, you are off the hook. You don't have to badger your client, or even ever talk about it again-you have fulfilled your duty. Additionally, you will feel better about yourself for having followed through with giving a professional recommendation rather than letting the concerns build up inside of you.

"No psychologist should pretend to understand what he does not understand... Only fools and charlatans know everything and understand nothing."

Anton Chekhov

Chapter 15

Memberships vs. Personal Training
Friends in evil places

The Membership Department

Gym memberships are the backbone to every gym in town. The monthly revenue obtained by memberships is what pays the salaries of the employees and the overhead of most facilities.

In most membership packages, they offer some type of discounted personal training package for the new member. Occasionally, the membership representative will sell a membership with the personal training sessions that you will service within. You will still get paid for the sessions serviced, though usually at a reduced rate and you will not see any commission from the original sale as that will go to the membership representative.

It is in your best interest to be friendly with the membership representatives and have a great rapport with them. They *will* be a source of revenue for you and snubbing these employees is like shooting yourself in the foot. There are always personality differences between membership representatives and personal trainers-it just *is*. You must look beyond your ego, and through any ego presented by an arrogant or stubborn membership representative.

Personal trainers tend to think they are *above* membership representatives in general, and this is to both the detriment of the gym and your personal training department. It is best to have a cohesive and smooth working environment with the membership and sales department. This can be obtained by going to lunch with the membership representatives and the sales manager, or by simply listening to them when you talk with them. Treat them as you would one of your clients; with respect, dignity, and value. This simple, yet seemingly difficult, task will make you a better trainer and open up doors for you that otherwise would be sealed shut.

The Personal Training Department

Personal trainers rule the gym floor. It's the nature of the beast. Yes, the general manager, sales manager, and the fitness manager will be high atop the cliffs with their eagle eyes ensuring that the operation runs smoothly; however, it is the personal trainer that is ruler.

Personal trainers are viewed as the experts on the floor. While the members are flailing about trying to decide what machine to go to and workout wrong on next (unintentionally, of course) trainers are giving guidance and unsolicited advice to their clients and members alike. If anyone has a question about a machine or a technique they do not go the general manager, they go to a personal trainer. If they somehow end up in front of the general manager, the general manager will call a personal trainer in to handle the member inquiry.

Most personal trainers have not only their national certifications, but also additional life experiences, athletic accomplishments, and higher education-more so than most membership representatives. This may be one of the factors causing the natural friction that comes between the personal training departments and membership/sales departments.

One of the best ways for you to earn the respect of the membership department and the sales manager is in public view on the exercise floor. After recognizing the strengths of any particular membership representative or of the sales manager, give them props by talking with a member about how good so and so is with _____ (fill in the blank.) This *will* get back to them, even if they are not in your presence. In contrast, raising gossip about the membership representatives or the sales manager will do the absolute opposite and cause for a strained working environment for you. Never speak ill of another employee inside of the gym or outside of the gym. If you must vent, do so with your companion or friends that do not have an interest in the gym. If you do otherwise, you will be hurting yourself and your client list will not grow like it should.

As a personal trainer, a salesman, you would be best served learning the membership sales process, fees, and subtleties. Once hired, inquire during non-peak hours to the sales manager, the general manager, and/or the membership representatives as to "how to" sell a membership. Learn the process. When the time comes for you to sell a membership, you will earn the commission and you can directly set that new member up for their personal training introduction. Additionally, there will be times when the gym becomes so busy that you will be able *to help* the membership representatives out when you are not occupied. There is no better way to get on the good graces of the sales department than to help them out in a bind.

Take the time as an intelligent and professional personal trainer to get to know the membership nuances and staff; you will be better for it.

"Business is not just doing deals; business is having great products, doing great engineering, and providing tremendous service to customers. Finally, business is a cobweb of human relationships."

Ross Perot

Chapter 16

Tangible Motivation:
Body fat tests: electronic impedance, calipers, Hydrostatic Weighing,
DEXA, & Bod Pod. Cloth tape measurements, Photographs
Efficiency compounded

One of the best ways for you to monitor your client's success will be through tracking their body fat %. That said, you will be hard pressed to use either the electronic devices or the hand held calipers to begin an accurate assessment for anyone over 30% body fat. The reason is obvious: there is too much body fat for you to accurately grab the intra-abdominal fat with the calipers, and the electronic devices have too much of a degree of inaccuracy for people over 30% body fat.

How do you, then, monitor your client's body fat %? You begin by taking an electronic impedance device body fat test like that of an Omron hand-held device. You will *know* beforehand if your client will exceed 30% body fat by your visual identification of how much extra body weight they are carrying.

I know this sounds contradicting, but you must give the visual tangible % to your client and then explain why the device will not be an accurate method to use for them. This may sound mean, but it isn't. Many people do not realize how truly obese they are and you are the exercise expert. Sure, their doctor will tell them that they are overweight, obese or fat, but hearing it from the exercise professional has a motivating element to it: *You are there to help them get fit*!

• **Electronic impedance devices**

There are a handful of available electronic apparatuses to measure one's body fat %. There are the at-home Tanita types of scales that are used commonly, and there are the Omron hand-held portable devices that can be found at places like Walgreens and online. The manuals claim to be within 3% of accuracy when compared to body fat calipers.

The devices *can* be accurate for some people-but the accuracy varies greatly. When using these devices hydration is a key factor. A dehydrated individual can measure significantly different than if they were hydrated. The harmless electronic pulse is dependent on water in your body for transference. The device works on the fact that body fat does not retain water like muscle will and so when the assessment is complete a certain body fat % is allocated for its result. It is critical that a person maintain the same hydration status at every measurement for accuracy. A typical recommendation is to take the measurement right after awakening and stepping out of bed. Food ingested, water consumed, sweat perspired, and alcohol consumed can all be factors in the inaccuracy of an electronic device.

Furthermore, if you have a woman that has a size D cup or larger breast size, the device can be way off as to the actual percentage of your client's body fat. Breast tissue is body fat. Imagine that you have a female client that looks like she is a magazine natural bodybuilding fitness model. Now imagine that you have to tell her that she has a body fat percentage of over 30%! That happened to me when I was a new trainer and it took me a few weeks of research and speaking with top doctors across the nation to find out the science behind those results. Needless to say, both my client and I laughed at the results. Ultimately, I measured that client's body fat via body fat calipers and deduced that her body fat was 20%. It could have been an uncomfortable situation, however, and it is a scenario I wish to spare you from experiencing.

Use the electronic devices to give your clients something to reference, with caution. For your clinically obese clients, use the device only when you are certain their body fat loss will provide them with motivation. Many clinically obese clients won't even register on an electronic device; it simply will give the result as an error message-try explaining *that* to your new client. This is usually the case when the person's body fat percentage is over 40%.

Electronic devices tend to work best when a person is between 5%-25% body fat, breast tissue notwithstanding.

- **Body fat calipers - skin fold measurements**

The use of body fat calipers is both time efficient and cost effective. Exercise physiologists and experts in exercise routinely use this method to monitor their client's body fat. The American College of Sports Medicine (ACSM) says that when performed by a trained & skilled tester, they are up to 98% accurate. You don't need a $200 body fat caliper either. A $10 body fat caliper will give you dependable measurements every time. You should begin right away as a new trainer by learning this method. The more you take body fat measurements, the more skilled you become. Your clients deserve an expert, give them one. Solicit the advice of the seasoned trainers at your new gym-they will be happy to guide you provided their egos are not too big.

- **Underwater - Hydrostatic Weighing**

Long held to be the gold standard for body fat assessment, the underwater method is on its way out like cassette tapes were in the 1990's. Newer assessments are being created that are not as time consuming or cumbersome as this process. There are a few hydrostatic weighing facilities around, but unless your client is an athlete that needs to closely monitor his body fat percentage for competition, it's a waste of time and money.

- **DEXA scan**

DEXA is the acronym for dual energy x-ray absorptiometry. The scan takes about fifteen minutes and costs around $100. The availability of this device is sporadic at best. You will have to search your area to find the closest one to you. This method is accurate with an approximate degree of error of only 3 percent, similar to the body fat calipers.

Again, unless you have an athlete who needs to closely monitor their body fat percentage, this device really is not a necessary one to use, but it *is* available.

- **Bod Pod**

The Bod Pod was introduced in 1994. Further developments were instituted by the company in 2002, 2004, and 2007. The Bod Pod has been used by the United States military and NFL teams, among other high profile users.

The Bod Pod is an "Air Displacement Plethysmograph which uses whole-body densitometry to determine body composition (fat and fat-free mass) in adults and children." http://www.bodpod.com/products/overviewBodpod

The Bod Pod seems to be a more realistic and practical approach compared to other premium body fat testing methods like the DEXA and Hydrostatic Weighing. Again, however, the need for a Bod Pod versus simply using the convenient body fat calipers is debatable. The Bod Pod presumably is the "new" gold standard compared to Hydrostatic Weighing in our current day and age with an amazingly reported 2% degree of accuracy.

- **Cloth tape measurements**

Clearly, cloth tape body measurements will not give you a body fat percentage. What the measurements will do is provide you with an accurate assessment for monitoring your client's progress. Like the body fat calipers, you must repeatedly take consistent cloth tape measurements of your clients to become skilled and accurate. These basic cloth tapes can be purchased at your local fabric store for only a few dollars.

The affordability and ease of use make cloth tape measurements a sure winner as one of the tools on your personal training tool belt. Keep one in your bag, one in your vehicle, and one in your work drawer or closet for quick and easy access.

There are two main reasons for taking both your client's body fat percentage and their body measurements. One is to give your client an accurate progress report to identify their results and the other is to supply excitement and motivation.

Your client will presumably already be having a good time with you and be feeling better by the time you revisit their body measurements and body fat %. Obtaining goals and getting results will keep your clients on your roster. They will in turn provide you with clients via references. If you do not include body fat assessments or cloth tape measurements, you will be limiting your effectiveness as a professional personal trainer.

- **Photographs: before, during and after photos**

A great motivational tool that you can use is to take before and after photos of your clients. Some clients are too embarrassed to take photographs, however, and you must be sensitive to their wants. You may elect to not use photographs as one of your motivating tools.

Personal trainers can be afraid to ask to take their clients' *before* and *after* photographs too! If you cringe at the thought of asking to take *before* and *after* photographs of your clients, you must obtain courage and get over your fear.

In the beginning, excessively obese clients are always full of self-doubt and embarrassment. After consistently being guided by you for four weeks, two months, and more, though, their confidence will shine like the sun. If they have *before* photographs to identify where they came from, they will be psychologically affected in a positive manner that will aid them in maintaining their weight loss.

If your clients do not have those photographs, their mind will not accurately recall how much of a difference they actually made. Make every effort to use the visual aid of photos at every opportunity that you can.

When you take these photographs, ask your client's permission to use their success story and photographs as motivation for future clients that come to you for help. They will tell you ok and sign the release document that you provide for them. This is an important marketing tool that you will be able to use for your entire career as a professional personal trainer. Begin to build your "book" now and ask every client that hires you as their trainer to do these *before* and *after* photos. This will also identify the confidence that you have in your client, as their trainer, and help prove to them that what you are preaching is possible. You, in effect, give them power and positive leverage by doing this.

"To keep the body in good health is a duty... otherwise we shall not be able to keep our mind strong and clear."

Buddha

Chapter 17

Science vs. Experience
Books and smiles

- **Science**

Your education in fitness will come from a source. This source may be one or a combination of the following: high school, community college, university, an Ivy League University, or simply a national personal training certification. Whatever your background, your education will form the foundation from which you will build and from which you will gain professional credibility in the fitness industry. You certainly do not need to have a college degree to be a top trainer, but it certainly will help.

- **Experience**

You can only gain hands-on training experience by application. You must train clients in order to gain the knowledge of all the subtleties and nuances that are found in the minor & major physical and psychological differences of people, in addition to their unique DNA compositions. You can earn every degree by every university, and you can earn every national certification by every national certifying body available; and not any of those will equal what you will gain by one-on-one training experience as the trainer.

As a hiring manager, I would prefer to entertain the application of a prospective employee that has experience with interaction of clients, rather than someone that has only a list of degrees identifying their clinical knowledge. This does not mean that I don't want both, I do. This only identifies the importance of training experience and contrasts it against the actual worth of a certification or degree. This is why it is important that you find a certification that fits your unique desires and passions. The better fitting certification will exploit your strengths, not work against them.

• The Real World

If you are an exercise physiologist with an advanced degree, you will be best served to obtain a national certification and to seek employment as a manager or director of operations for exercise at an institution or within a clinical setting. Exercise physiologists tend to have an air of superiority about them that doesn't work well in a personal training team atmosphere. Too much education can work against a person in the personal training industry.

People want to work with charismatic, fun, intelligent and inspiring individuals. They do not want to spend hours and hours with a non-emotional professor dictating what they must do and how many. There are exceptions, of course, and I'm certainly not advocating that you avoid an education as an exercise physiologist. Exercise physiologists are some of the most anal people around when it comes to being correct and doing the right thing. These are traits that I would like to see when it comes to personal trainers, in general.

The main difference between exercise physiologists and professional personal trainers is that the exercise physiologist typically has a background of experience in a clinical setting. The professional personal trainer, on the other hand, has life experience and thousands of real encounters with clients in the private industry of a gym setting. There are a few exercise physiologists that survive and thrive as professional personal trainers and become successful at opening up their own personal training studios, but they are few and far between.

As a professional personal trainer, you are taxed with the responsibility of balancing your education and your science, along with your experience training one-on-one. It is important that you carry a nice combination of both in order to identify with well-educated clients that will be CEO's, doctors, attorneys and the like. If you cannot communicate intelligently with your higher education clients, you will not be effective with them in their training program and you will lose those clients. To be a successful professional personal trainer, you must be a chameleon and work well with all types of people with various educational backgrounds.

"Science, at bottom, is really anti-intellectual. It always distrusts pure reason, and demands the production of objective fact."

Henry Louis Mencken

Chapter 18

Professional stretches, PNF, AIS
The money maker

There are two dominant professional stretches used today by exercise professionals for their clients and for their Pro teams: NFL, NBA, NHL, MLB & US Soccer. These stretching methods are: proprioceptive neuromuscular facilitation (PNF) & active isolated stretching (AIS).

There are similarities between both the PNF and AIS methods. You can find books on each method online and at your local bookstore.

As a professional personal trainer, you must add to your tool belt of knowledge and experience in order to further your strengths, and to remain competitive in a highly competitive market. If you learn either the PNF or the AIS approach to flexibility, you will enhance your clients' experience beyond your wildest imagination.

Every client that you perform these Pro stretches with will be thankful for your application of them. Implementing these stretches into your client's workout can also be the difference between successfully selling a personal training package to them and not selling them sessions.

The application of PNF or AIS will both increase your retention of clients, and make your clients feel better. With as little as ten minutes at the end of your client's session, you can touch them in an almost spiritual manner without even trying to.

Take the time to learn either PNF or AIS and practice the methods learned frequently. Some corporate gyms do offer training by an instructor in these methods for a fee. If you can find an instructor to teach you PNF or AIS, take the class! I don't care if the class is $50 or $200, you *want* this training! You can alternatively purchase the clinical books online, as mentioned, but there really is not a substitution for learning from an instructor that has performed these stretches hundreds, if not thousands, of times on clients.

- Note: Science has not identified a clear winner or optimal stretching method, yet, when it comes to flexibility training. There is a reason that the Pros use these stretches and it's simple-*they work*!

"...having lived long, I have experienced many instances of being obliged by better information, or fuller consideration, to change opinions even on important subjects, which I once thought right, but found to be otherwise. It is therefore that the older I grow, the more apt I am to doubt my own judgment, and to pay more respect to the judgment of others."

Ben Franklin

Chapter 19

Group EX
(The classes, the instructors, the participants)
A league of their own

Group exercise is the second most visible activity occurring in a gym. Personal trainers attending their clients is the first most identifiable activity, outside of members using the machines by themselves, of course.

Group exercise instructors are in a league of their own. They teach everything from dance aerobics to kickboxing and they even offer blanket weight training classes now too. Most of these nationally certified aerobics instructors thrive on teaching in a class environment. These classes have as many as thirty or more participants.

Some of the most successful personal trainers also teach classes on the group exercise schedule. These classes are usually something like: abs, cardio-kickboxing, ab-aerobics, and boot camps. The personal trainers that offer these classes always end up obtaining a few personal training clients from participants in these classes, in the long run. This is the reason that they teach the classes: They know that they will receive additional exposure. This exposure is to gym members that ordinarily would never approach a personal trainer for advice and would shrug off any attempt by a personal trainer to sell them training. In effect, it is a way to create some of your personal training business and give great service to gym members.

The pay received for your time, however, pales in comparison to what you will receive training your clients one-on-one in personal training. You may only receive minimum wage for teaching a group class, which can be exhausting. In some instances, you may make up to $20 per class. Consider the fact that personal trainers are looking to make $25-45 per hour for every personal training session that they service; and you can easily identify why personal trainers prefer to train vs. give group exercise classes.

Group exercise instructors, and group exercise managers, are always on the go. They have other jobs and they travel from gym to gym servicing different classes and covering for instructors that have to cancel for one reason or another. Group exercise instructors don't have to sell their classes, they just show up and teach. This is one of the greatest draws to becoming a group exercise instructor against that of a personal trainer: they don't have to sell anything, they teach. The fear of being a salesman, or the lack of a desire to be one, is one of the main differences between the two careers.

Personal trainers and group exercise instructors march to different drummers, as a whole. Arguably, professional personal trainers are there to make a career out of their work and group exercise instructors seek to add to their lives by teaching exercise classes part-time.

Many participants in group exercise are members of the gym *solely* for the ability to attend these group classes! Have you ever been in a gym working out and right before a group class begins you see a mad exodus of people coming from the entrance doors and heading directly to the large group exercise room? Then, promptly upon the class termination, you see the same herd fly out the door! This is important to recognize as a professional personal trainer trying to fill your schedule with clients. You can become a participant yourself in these classes to indirectly meet these members. It's a sales method that I call "indirect sales." Or, as mentioned, you can teach a class and meet the members directly.

A lot of personal trainers completely dismiss the potential and the use of the group exercise schedule. You can go into any gym and ask any personal trainer the names of the group exercise instructors at *their* gym and learn promptly that they don't know.

Similar to getting to know the sales staff, it is equally important for you to make an effort to get to know every aerobics instructor in the building. The common statement made by trainers regarding this is, "They don't last long enough for me to get to know their name." That is ridiculous and just plain lazy.

You are looking to build a positive work atmosphere and full client base as a professional personal trainer. You must work at building your client list; it will not come simply because of your presence. The group exercise facet of any gym will add to your repertoire, if you allow it to.

"I have to exercise in the morning before my brain figures out what I'm doing."

Marsha Doble

Chapter 20

Pilates & Yoga
(The instructors and the participants; a unique group)
The rare entities

Pilates and yoga instructors are the polar opposite of group exercise instructors, generally. You will find these teachers taking time to get to know their students and off in a corner talking about holistic remedies or approaches to life. They are on their own timeline and are ninja! They slip in and they slip out of the gym without much notice.

If you plan ahead, you can catch these great people while they are setting up the room for their class. You can take one of their classes, too, of course. Either way, you must not exclude the importance of getting to know these instructors. They are a genuine bunch of good people that will direct business your way, if they believe in your confidence and abilities.

The best approach for you with Pilates and yoga instructors is to be genuine. Find real reasons for you to get to know them; not artificial excuses. If you tell them directly that you only want to know them for referrals, you probably won't get any. These instructors have a connection with their "followers" and if you are not sincere, you simply will not get business from them.

The participants of Pilates and yoga are rare. They definitely march to the beat of a different drummer compared to anyone else in the facility. The managers will refer to the Pilates and yoga clan as "those guys" or "that group" in an almost derogatory manner. Of course, these managers will put on a front and be helpful for anyone involved with Pilates or yoga, but the fact of the matter is that the managers generally don't understand the plight of the Pilates or yoga participants. Many of the Pilates and yoga participants believe that their activities are a panacea of sorts. I won't get into the science or psychology here, just know that these teachers and students are good and sincere individuals. As a professional looking to expand your business, you can also benefit from not excluding these groups within the gym, which is usually what trainers do.

"I've been using Pilates for many years. It's the best system I've found for isolating and strengthening individual muscles without stress to the joints."

Patrick Swayze

Chapter 21

Men vs. Women in Personal Training
(Who makes a better or more successful trainer?)
Mars & Venus

Who make better trainers: men or women? What gender makes for a more successful trainer? Men and women alike can be equally successful. What determines whether or not a person will be successful as a professional personal trainer is not the person's sex. It is the fulfillment of their potential. There are, however, some easily observable differences in clientele between the different genders.

For example, if there is a male trainer that looks like a cover of Muscle & Fitness, this personal trainer will attract men that want to bulk up, without having to market himself or obtain referrals. He simply obtains clients because of the fallacy that people believe he must know what he is doing if he looks like that. The women that tend to sign up with these muscle bound trainers are very fit themselves-most want to compete in the bodybuilding world or are a part of a competitive circuit of some kind.

A slender young college aged female trainer, in contrast, will be approached by middle-aged women who want to look like them and by men who just want to be trained by a pretty woman. They will not have to market themselves much either, they will get business simply *because* of the way they look.

In both of these examples, *looks* are what determines a large portion of the clientele received by those trainers. It may seem ridiculous, which it is, but it's true.

The rest of the "normal" looking trainers, male and female, have to fight for each client that they get by giving great service, and by getting referrals.

Success as a trainer, male or female, is dependent on several factors. You must have personality. You must have charisma. You must have communication skills. You must be a good listener. You must be able to teach. You must be professional. You must be able to scientifically explain yourself when needed, or at least bluff. You must be on-time for your session, every time. You must be a leader. You must have confidence. You must have courage. You must safely guide your client in an exercise program that gets results. You must smell good. You must keep your hygiene above average-no bad breath! You must *give* of yourself to your client for every minute of their session-pay attention!

The only way to recognize an injury before it occurs is to be able to *"feel"* what your client is doing and where they are at during every repetition and every set. If you have it in your head that you told your client to do fifteen repetitions, so you will be damned if they do less, you will injure your client and be out of a job lickity-split! Similarly, if you are leaning on a machine, and talking to the pretty girl or handsome guy elsewhere, you do not deserve to be training that client-go home. There is also no reason for you to be talking to the other trainers or employees, regardless of how popular you might be. Your client paid you to pay attention to them and to train them-it is your responsibility to do just that.

Tunnel vision is usually something to turn away from. This is the one exception: With your client! You must make every session for every client one that is a dynamic and enriching experience. Treat every session like it is your interview for your job, and you will begin to understand how important every session is to your client. It's easy to overlook the importance you have in their life as their trainer. Always keep this in the back of your mind: "I'm training this person for $100 per hour! How would I like to be treated if I were paying $100 per hour for service?" Sure you may only be making $25 for that session, but the same principle applies.

The differences between men and women personal trainers are as unique as we are people. Your success depends on you, not your gender.

"Why are women so much more interesting to men than men are to women?"

Virginia Woolf

Chapter 22

Biggest Loser & 24 hour fitness training mentality
Insanity + danger = motivation

The television reality series *The Biggest Loser* became an overnight success with Bob and Jillian heading the red and blue teams into the air waves. The training philosophy, from the beginning, was geared toward entertainment value, not toward the enrichment of peoples' lives. If there was some life enriching along the way, so be it, was their frame of mind.

It wasn't the dream of changing lives and inspiring millions of people to become fit that brought this show to the main stage. It was money, of course. What brought this reality show into mainstream popularity, on the other hand were the drastic and seemingly impossible feats of losing rapid amounts of weight fast.

We also saw the good cop/bad cop portrayed very well by Bob and Jillian, the 24 Hour Fitness trainers. It's ironic that these two trainers have been portrayed as America's Fitness Experts when the reality is that *The Biggest Loser* is about ratings, not about weight loss and positive changes in people's lives.

The personal training philosophy of Bob and Jillian may never be really known. What we do know is what *The Biggest Loser* show, sponsored by 24 Hour Fitness, advertised as the best way to lose significant amounts of body weight. They consistently beat up their contestants and pushed their bodies to their real limits. These limits were real and beyond what their body should have undergone for a safe and effective weight loss program. The amount of pressure placed on their knees, for example, during a marathon that finished on the beach for those contestants over

300 pounds is mind boggling. If you want lifetime damage to your knees and you weigh over 300 pounds, the clear way to get damage is to run a marathon and then finish in the sand on a beach.

The purpose of giving you that example is to show you how ludicrous *The Biggest Loser* program had become. They keep pushing the limit of peoples' abilities, and breaking safety rules all along the way, simply to get ratings. This author got so disgusted at yelling at the television that after the senior citizen got hurt and transported to the hospital, I stopped watching. I only wish that Bob or Jillian had quit the show in protest, after becoming successful, for what they were being forced to do with the participants. I'm sure these trainers had to sign some type of clause in their contract, however, that precluded them from bad-mouthing the show or that of 24 Hour Fitness. I would like to get these trainers in private and give them a real talking to.

The positive impact of *The Biggest Loser*, though, cannot be overlooked. Scores of individuals that ordinarily would not have begun an exercise program did just that; they began to exercise! This is a dilemma: Have clinically obese people remain at home and *not* be motivated to take action to exercise and become healthier; or slaughter a ton of individuals who voluntarily put their heads on a chopping block, which then becomes the catalyst for these clinically obese people to lose weight, from a show like *The Biggest Loser*? Since these people volunteered, I have to say that they did not make an intelligent choice, but okay. I will accept their sacrifice for the benefit of millions, but what a price to pay!

I worked with a television producer for a short period of time that was beginning a *Biggest Loser* type of show with the motto, "Putting the *reality* back into reality television!" His premise and ideas were sound. The reality, though, was that he couldn't obtain the financial support to continue his vision and his program fizzled. Without putting people into harm's way, the television appeal was not present.

As a professional personal trainer it is your duty, no, it is your *obligation* to enhance the fitness industry in a positive fashion and to provide great, fun, and safe service to your clients. Do not take *The Biggest Loser* approach to fitness and treat everyone like they fit into a professional athlete cookie-cutter. If you do, you will have injured clients and lawsuits. *The Biggest Loser* has high powered attorneys and can afford to pay off anyone that sues them-you do not.

"Genius has no youth, but starts with the ripeness of age and old experience."

Mark Twain

Chapter 23

Firing a client
When it's time for the cows to go home

There will come a time, *or two*, that during your career as a personal trainer you will have a client on your roster that is not a pleasure for you to work with. Rather, it's a chore. You may have had red flags initially that you simply dismissed or perhaps you knew it wouldn't be the best working relationship, but maybe you needed the money.

Whether you initiate the conflict, or your client initiates the static, the time will surface when you decide that you will no longer tolerate the behavior of your client. What do you do? You fire them.

Once you have decided that you must fire your client, be swift. Take immediate action! Write down all of the positive traits (dig deep!) about that client on a sheet of paper for your own reference.

If you are self-employed, write up a referral for them to take that they can present to their new trainer. The referral should be a professional written clinical evaluation of your work with this client and it should contain all of the specific strength and conditioning aspects of your client's progression. You can include your name and contact information for the new trainer, as well. If you are contacted by the new trainer, do not bad mouth your client. Simply state that you had a personality conflict with this client and that you felt they would be better suited training with another trainer for a better fit and for their benefit. This is part of what you want to tell your client when you inform them that you will be parting ways with them.

If you are employed by a gym, speak with the personal training manager immediately. Sit down with him and be honest. Explain to him what the situation is and that you will not be able to continue with that client. By this time, you will most likely know the other trainers' training styles and attitudes pretty well. You can mention to the manager who you think might work best with this client, and why, but leave the whole decision process up to your manager. The manager may even elect to handle the "firing" for you by sitting down with your client and offering a free session or two with one or two of the other trainers on the floor until they select one. In this way, your client not only keeps the sessions that they have remaining from their training package, but they also will not feel as jilted. People tend to take getting fired as a client as a slap in the face. They feel that *they* hired you, and what right do you have to fire them?

Of course, you will not talk to your client at all like that. You will not be Donald Trump and say, "You're fired!" Instead, you will be diplomatic and professional. You will sit down with your client and tell them that after assessing their progression up until this point, you feel that they would be a better fit for another trainer. You will inform them that as an expert in the exercise industry, you recognize when the working relationship is not as smooth as it should be. You tell them that you want the best possible outcome for them and for the resources that they have spent, and therefore it's in their best interest to train with another trainer. Then, you inform them that you will either return their money (if you are self-employed) or that your manager will sit down with them so that they can make another selection for a personal trainer.

Your client may ask you for a trainer recommendation, and you should be prepared to answer this question along with the question, why? Though you have fully explained yourself, they may still be in a sort of shock and need further explanation. You will have to give them different information to satisfy their intellect. You will then tell them that while your experience is vast and your knowledge is good, that you believe a better customized program can be achieved from another trainer that has a fresh perspective on their desires and goals.

Sure, you can tell them, "Hey, I can't work with you! You're fired! You are such a whiner and cry baby!" But, that will not go over too well with them, your manager, or with your other clients that *will* catch wind of what happened. When your other clients ask you what happened, also, it is your duty to remain tight lipped, regardless of how close you are to those clients. You must remain professional and not gossip. Your answer to anyone who asks must be only to the effect of, "Sometimes it happens in personal training that a trainer and their client are not a great fit. I felt that they were better suited for another trainer and I wish them well."

A personal example: Several years ago, I had trained an individual for a few months. They had paid over 3k up front for training with me. I had been to this client's home, in addition to training them at my studio. This client was extremely difficult to manage as they were a hypochondriac and had personal issues that were way beyond my scope of duty. Since this person was extremely intelligent, and wealthy, they would have been beyond offended had I told them I felt they needed to see a psychologist. I did confer with this client's doctor, however, and I had previous permission to share information with this doctor from this client.

I chose the high road and had a meeting with this client. I told them that their program was not progressing the way that it should, largely in part because they would not execute my recommendations outside of the gym, and that their efforts were less than 100% while in the gym. I told this client that I would not work with them any longer; however, I would give names of two or three other trainers that they might be interested in working with.

The client was offended and in defense raised the fact that they had paid so much money for the training and that they had selected me as their trainer and they didn't want anybody else. I apologized and told them that as their professional personal trainer, the exercise expert, that it was my conclusion that they would be better suited with another trainer that was a better fit for them, for *their* benefit. I quenched their complaint about paying money by telling them I was giving them a full refund of the 3k+ that they had paid up front for my services. This resulted in a pleasant moment of silence. Even though I had already serviced two months of agonizing sessions with this individual, it was worth it to give this client a full refund.

Sometimes, it is best to sever ties completely, even if it means taking a little bit of a loss financially. Sure, I could have taken out my calculator and subtracted my fees for the sessions that I had serviced, and I would have been legally in the right to do just that. Believe me, I *wanted* to! Not for the money though, it was the principle of the matter and having to work with such a difficult client for so long was worth about 10 times what I had been paid. Yet, there I was returning all of the money *and* giving two months of free service. Believe me; it was *worth* it to be rid of this client once and for all. Had I deducted sessions for the work already performed, you can bet that this client would have complained incessantly and I may even have had to go to court, not to mention the repercussions from my other clients hearing rumors.

When you recognize it is time to fire a client, be expeditious-do not prolong the pain. Be courteous, professional, and direct. Do not waver. *You* are the exercise professional. *You* get to decide who you work with. Your clients may believe that they selected you, and that's ok, let them continue to believe that.

- Manager's note: You are in the leadership position and in control of your gym's personal training business. You must take the time to stroke the ego of a client that has been fired by their trainer. This may even entail you taking over this client as one of your own. Be empathetic and dismiss the occurrence as one of familiarity, though you may never have had to experience a client getting fired before, you must act like it is not a big deal and that it happens from time to time. You can add credence to your trainer's action and give the client satisfaction both at the same time by stating, "I had a feeling that you were not a good match for that trainer, but I was going to give it a few more weeks to see if it was going to work out for you." Then, you can segue into, "I was thinking "Joe" would be a good fit for you, would you like to try two free sessions on me with "Joe" to see if he will meet your expectations?"

- The client may say no, and mention the name of another trainer that they might like to work with. Either way, you win. The client has begun the acceptance of moving on and training with another trainer. If the client is completely destroyed from the experience, they may demand a refund. Gyms typically have clauses that the client has signed stating that they will not get a refund, I know. In the case of a belligerent client, you may have to console them and offer them a few of the freebies that you as the manager of the gym can offer. Or, you may simply have to get the general manager involved to resolve the conflict. Most often, you will never have to get to this point if you and your trainer are calm, empathetic, diplomatic, *and* offering free service or goodies. Whatever you have to do to make this client happy, do it. If you don't, the gym and your whole department will suffer the after effects for an indefinite period of time, unless the member is so disruptive that you completely ban them from the gym, that is.

"Never continue in a job you don't enjoy. If you're happy in what you're doing, you'll like yourself, you'll have inner peace. And if you have that, along with physical health, you will have had more success than you could possibly have imagined."

Johnny Carson

Chapter 24

When a client discontinues training
(The best protocol to follow with them)
Positive separation

As a successful professional personal trainer, you will have the rare occurrence of parting ways with one of your great clients. You are accustomed to retaining your clients indefinitely and when a client informs you that they cannot continue training for whatever reason, you must be prepared to handle their departure in a pleasant and skilled manner.

The odds are that your client has been dwelling over this need of theirs and this decision for weeks. You will need to be gentle in your acceptance of their decision to cease to train with you. They will give you their reasons as to why this need has arisen, and they will be sad about it. You have been their wonderful trainer for years, in most instances, and losing your regular weekly interaction will be tantamount to attending the funeral of a loved one for them.

You can ease the tension for your client by being extremely sensitive and empathetic. Offer to give them a few free sessions, perhaps one per week for two or three weeks to help with the transition into working out by themselves. They will have questions and they will need your support and guidance. If you do not do this, they may fall off the face of the earth and stop exercising all together. You can further ease this transition for them by ensuring you keep email and/or phone contact with them on the regular days that you normally would train with them. For all of the money that they have paid to train with you, not to mention the friendship that has arisen, this is the *least* that you can do for them! Do not consider this a nuisance, consider it a privilege.

You will find, in the long run, when you make the extra effort and take the time for your client to depart training with you in a comfortable and pleasant manner, that they will one day return for training with you, or that you will get several additional referrals from them. This has been a great working relationship and when they see how you treat them after they leave, they will be motivated to promote you to others that they know because they want their friends to have both a great trainer and a good experience too.

in omnia paratus: **Prepared for all things.**

Chapter 25

Conclusion
You are worthy

You can be a successful professional personal trainer. You can make over $100,000 per year in gross income and own your own personal training studio and equipment. You can work as few as twenty hours per week and make a comfortable living, or you can work as many as 40 or 50 hours per week and push the threshold of your income to its highest potential.

Whether you are a successful expert in the fitness industry, or you fizzle out after a short few months, it is completely dependent on you. If you follow the examples, ideas, and professional approaches outlined in this book, you will be successful. If you don't, and you just throw on a personal trainer's t-shirt and expect people to play to your ego, you might as well start looking for another job or career right now.

The methods and experiences that you have now become aware of are tried and true methods in the real world. This is the reality of being a personal trainer. This is not a text book on how to get a certification and how to get a job and follow the strict advice of whatever national certifying entity, this is a how-to-be-successful guide for anyone that wants to be a top trainer and fitness expert; while making a good salary and looking out for your best interests along the way.

Follow the spirit of this book and you will have a great retirement. You will also have all of the critical components that come with being a personal trainer in demand and that have a waiting list of clients.

You have learned the skills, procedures, and the realities of the personal training industry all in the concise text of this book. I wish you the utmost success and happiness in the outstanding career of a professional personal trainer. Now, put on your happy face, get motivated & inspired, and go train!

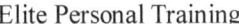

"We don't grow unless we take risks. Any successful company is riddled with failures."

James E. Burke

My utmost gratitude is extended to you for taking the time to read my book. Thank you for your attention and time in space. I wish you the greatest success of your mind's eye!

~ Dwayne D. Ivey

Author Biography

Dwayne Ivey is an expert in Kenpo Karate & Sports Therapy. He began teaching Kenpo in 1999 and soon thereafter began personal training. He successfully managed the personal training departments of major health clubs in Phoenix, Arizona, for several years.

In 2007, he began his own successful business as a Clinical Exercise Specialist inside of a concierge doctor's medical office in Tucson, Arizona, where he remained for two years.

Dwayne Ivey has since maintained an elite clientele in both Kenpo Karate & Sports Therapy in three states, in addition to writing. He has traveled both internationally and domestically as an instructor in Kenpo Karate as well as domestically for Sports Therapy functions.

The media recently labeled Dwayne Ivey as a "Health Guru" due to his copious published critical write-ups on diets and weight loss.

Visit the author's website at: www.DwayneIvey.com

You may also contact the author at: ivey021@gmail.com

Please allow up to two weeks for a reply.

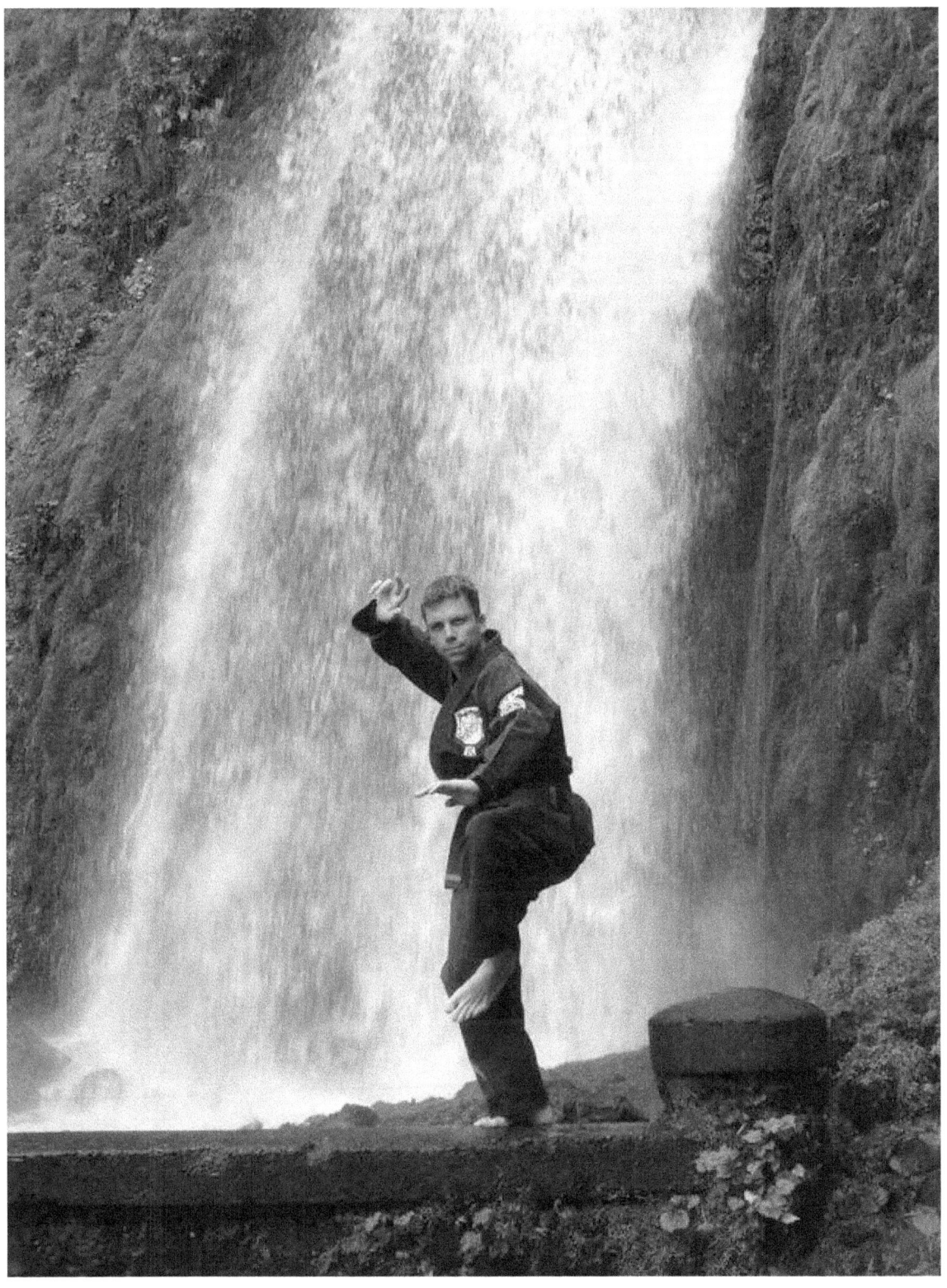